Twenty-five Days to Enlightenment

Alan Hoxie

2018

Hako had been studying under a great master to become enlightened, and asked him what he must do." Hako, he answered," You must demonstrate to me that you are a man of virtue and honor a man of your word, and a humble man. You must show me that you put service to others ahead of yourself and you must do the simplest chores with honor. You must chop wood and carry water."

  ---Do not seek Truth--- Simply let go of all Opinion--Buddha

  I sit here, the evening before my flight to San Jose, Costa Rica, hoping I have everything packed. Everything that I will need for my twenty-five day stay at the yoga retreat where I hope to earn my Yoga teaching certificate, sponsored by Yoga Alliance. I am going alone, and that is a good thing because climbing the ladder to enlightenment is not a tandem experience. The physical aspect of

Yoga {unity of mind and body}, is about certain postures done correctly and what muscle groups are involved in their execution. The other aspects of Yoga are not foreign to me and would be, to me, a challenge, I thought. I was not a novice at meditation, having done so since the 70's and have lead meditation groups at various times in my life. Was it part of my daily regimen? I must confess, no.

I will remain open to the teaching of the young woman who owned the Yoga retreat, and her assistants, and do what they say. After all at 67 years old it was time I became teachable. I think I will probably be among a gaggle of 26 year old, flexible female Millennial, but as I learned long ago, from my daughter of that age, I am no match for them, on any level. I also imagined there would be a few folks who had been taking yoga a year or so whose parents simply wanted them out of the house and they thought Yoga Teacher Training would be a good idea. I am going to give it a go to try and be vulnerable, open and teachable. All this is just a polite way of saying that as often as I can, I will keep my mouth shut.

Doing the Yoga didn't bother me so much. I had done several kinds of yoga over the years and I felt comfortable doing two classes per day for 20 days .I did not start Yoga until I was 50, but since then I had 5 years of Hatha,Vinyasa, with a little Astanga thrown in, and since moving to Arizona from New York, had completed just under 1600 Bikram Yoga classes, in 8 years, most of which were 90 minutes, in a 105 degree room. I had captured first place in the Senior Men's Division of the Arizona Regional Yoga competition 2014, with a routine I picked out of coffee table yoga books, and thought I could hold my own with these flexible whipper -snappers. I had just finished teacher training as a Yin Yoga instructor, so this was not my first rodeo. But could I keep from feeling my age on several fronts. We all hope we fit in and this was no exception for me. I had been doing doubles of one hour Yoga followed by another hour of Pilates, twice a week, for several months, in addition to yoga classes three times per week , to prepare, but one can never be sure especially when there is a significant change in humidity, as there will be when I land in Costa Rica.

The 6 hour direct flight from Phoenix was a bit bumpy but otherwise enjoyable until getting in the wrong line at customs and trying to negotiate the cab fare when I had no idea what was fair or customary. After negotiating a 20$ cab ride to my hotel on the west side of San Jose, which, as it turned out, was worth it since it was a twenty minute trip, I tipped him as well and dragged my bags inside the cute boutique hotel I found on line for 54 bucks a night. The next day after a fitful nights sleep due to the sound of locals settling of a few differences outside my window. I woke and had breakfast cooked by Ana who I immediately fell for, then I decided to go scouting for some shave cream to replace the can that TSA had taken from me for fear of me grabbing a stewardess and frothing her face with it unless I got another bag of pretzels on my bumpy plane ride. As I walked around I couldn't help notice that every property was fully fenced including the driveway and some had razor wire on the top of the fencing. It didn't look like a particularly bad neighborhood but this is a time when the feeling is, "if it ain't tied down it's mine." This attitude prevails in much of the world. Gone are the days of right and wrong. It was odd to see so much security around a simple residence, and wondered if there had been a social revolution here. I just wished I had the franchise for razor wire and padlocks.

After turning down offers of around ten dollars for a can of shave cream from a couple of local shops I finally rendered a deal at the AM/PM for 6 dollars for a can the size I could bring back on the plane, if there was any left.

On my way back to the hotel I couldn't help but notice the abundance of beautiful plants being ubiquitous. Most of them the type you'd want to buy for the indoors of your property and water graciously. From June to November it is common for this country to receive 10 inches or more per month in rainfall and it was evident. The hotel Casa Roland about 4 miles outside of San Jose is an eclectic old style place with all kinds of art work and nic- nacs tucked into corners and hung from ceilings. You would expect Humphrey Bogart to walk through the door at any minute. Dark wood trim everywhere, huge ceiling fans shaped like palm leaves. The place reminded me of Hotel Chelsea on 23rd St. in Manhattan where in the lobby is an erratic display of all of the art the owner had traded for a room over the years. Warhol prints on the wall next to original poetry by Dylan Thomas and other paraphernalia on display. Staying at The Roland was like staying in an art museum, I would stay there again in a heartbeat. Probably will on the way back.

-----People will soon forget what you've said, and sooner still what you've done, but they will never forget the way you made them feel------

I tried to remember that saying on this my second day in Costa Rica. I sit here in the lobby of the Roland waiting for a cab to take me back to the airport to catch a shuttle for the four hour drive to Uvita on the Pacific Coast, home to the Yoga school. I could see from my newly installed What's Up app that I would be meeting women with names like Courtney, Monica, Michelle, and Nikki, with two K's, Sidharra, Ziggy, and Tara. No matter what, I was going to keep my mouth shut, be vulnerable and open and free from judgment. This was a practice for me just like Yoga, because it did not come naturally. For years I had to be in control and know all the answers and be the bull goose, but the older I got, I realized that those ideas were born of fear and that I was not nominated or anointed to be this way. Being a know-it-all from a very early age made this hard for me, and it had been even more so in my drinking days, now 15 years behind me. I was going to enjoy the ride down the coast through beautiful towns like Dominica and Jaco and Uvita where we were staying. I had not known that much of the Pacific Coast of this country. It is a Mecca for surfers, Jaco having many Surf Hotels, on the ocean. Additionally Costa Rica is a Mecca for Yogis behind only a few ashrams in Rishikesh, India, at the foot of the Himalayas. That's why I decided to come here to be certified. When you train in Costa Rica, everyone in the Yoga world watches, and respects you. This would be the day we would all get settled in and begin classes, tomorrow, Monday. It would at least be a relief to abandon my three bags of luggage at a fixed address for three weeks before leaving after my graduation, of course, for which we were required to bring white clothing. I suppose that if someone didn't graduate they could always be sacrificed to some God, since they were already wearing white, or be married, but is there a difference?

Our shuttle ride from the Capital down the Pacific coast was typical third world. Two lane roads, dogs everywhere, we stopped twice, once to see crocodiles in the river below our van, and to look at free flying Macaws.

After an arduous 4 hour drive we reached our destination. It was good to be somewhere to hang my hat for a while after lugging around three bags of luggage. There were three guys and twelve women. A newly minted Doctor, Ray, a charming guy from North Carolina, who spoke fluent Spanish, and my roommate a supplement Guru and overall nice kid and me. Of course I was the oldest of the bunch, and kept quiet to hide my age. After all everyone knows old folks complain about everything. Here I had a chance to be twenty-something again, if I kept quiet. My body is in pretty good shape for my age but no one would NOT guess me for at least 50 yrs old. I was not going to judge myself. That was my Mantra.

A bunch of us hiked a few blocks to the main road to eat, and to my surprise a small outdoor restaurant had the Super bowl on. As we were ordering, a truck pulled up and dropped off an inflatable T. V. Screen, thirty foot by twenty, installed a projector on the deck and a PA system next to it. Bingo we were watching the Big Dance in a Soccer loving country, outdoors like going to the drive-ins. I didn't see the Eagles take down the Patriots, as I would have liked, since I was too tired. And anyway I didn't think Brady was capable of another comeback. We had to be up at 6 am for Yoga in the Jungle.

My bed was ok, a twin, and my roommate a nice kid, but the rooster that started at 3 am and kept it up, I could have strangled, had this not been a vegetarian place. The owner read us the ground rules no booze or drugs, or any meats or sugars on the property. This was also a detoxifying junket. She made us promise. We were informed that toilet paper used for any reason including number two, must be put in the trash, not flushed down the toilet. I'm not sure why this bothered me so much. I'm not a particularly fussy person, nor am I fastidious about cleanliness or my clothes, and have been known to wear underwear a number of days, providing they passed the smell test.

It's just that in this day and age of artificial intelligence, space travel, driverless cars, fake news being realer than real news, and an inordinate degree of interest in the bathroom habits of transsexuals, I find it hard to believe that NO ONE has invented toilet paper that dissolves as it touches the water. This thought haunted me for a few days, before other issues took precedence. A fortune is out there waiting to be made by some College of Forestry graduate. I go on record as claiming ten percent for lofting this melting toilet paper idea, in a public forum.

Our room was sparse, two twin beds, the outlet on my wall didn't work so I plugged my computer and phone charger in the bathroom. The faucet had to be held with two hands since it was not anchored at the sink. The water in Costa Rica was drinkable and actually quite good.

I set my phone for 5:30 and needed it to ring, to wake me up. I had set my yoga gear aside and was ready to go. I joined the line of Yogis walking to the platform to begin our morning session. The Leaf ants were already busy at work carrying huge chunks of leaves across the dirt and down into a huge hole. I had briefly met and had a small chat with most of the women that night.

It was really quite inspiring to set my mat, upside down, on the platform and get a good look at twelve beautiful young women that had come here from all over the world. I vowed to be a good friend to everyone and not another harasser worthy of a # Me Too, charge. I was here for a reason and nobody was interested in an ancient Yogi.

-----A man who can control his mind is mightier than he who controls vast armies.------

The morning of day one, we were, after breakfast, going to do some team building exercises and get better acquainted since we were to be together for 24 more days. The owner's husband was introduced as a former Eagle Scout and his father as a current scout leader in Pennsylvania. They had devised some team building exercises that scouts use on their campouts, you can't make this shit up! Immediately I panicked. How bizarre was this going to be if it was devised by these folks? Be careful what you wish for.. kept rolling through my head. I was the only male on my team and first we all had to pass our team members through a spider web of holes made by various rope knots. We passed each other through and back and I was careful to handle the merchandise with care. I was mostly the passer since I was the tallest. I tried to keep my hands in the right places. We were then placed on a four by four about 8 ft long and the goal was for the end person to make it to the other end, and back. Well I had to closely, hip to hip, hug most of the women to get beyond them. First the one from Sweden and then hang onto the waist of the one from Argentina, as I wriggled by Ziggie from Iceland. We were all pretty close along that beam but we succeeded in our goal. I was sweating from trying to think only pure thoughts, and was actually glad it was over. They seemed ok with the slow dance aspect of it and I tried my best not to think beyond holding them for the sake of the game, geeeze Louise! My yoga pants showed otherwise. It was, however, an ice breaker.

We visited the jungle platform where we practiced our asana's(yoga pose)as a group, at least twice a day and led small groups ourselves, right from the first day. Our teacher led us through what she called an Astanga warm-up. It was in fact ninety minutes of some of the hardest Yoga I had ever done. We must have done 15 vinyasa, plank, chaturunga, up dog, down dog, not my favorite grouping. I had been taking a specialty Yoga, Bikram, for 8 years and knew that someday that would bite me in the ass. This was that day. Bikram Yoga has 26 postures that never vary and don't include some of yogas' most popular asanas. Needless to say I was in bed by 8 ignoring my assigned homework. I got up, this second day, at 5:30 as I would every day but Saturday and Sunday. This day we were hiking to a nearby waterfall for a quick swim before going to our platform for morning Yoga. The rustle of tree tops nearby was clearly heard as we walked up the dirt road past the police station, and eagerly followed three white faced capuchin monkeys, chasing each other through the tree tops. They seemed not a bit interested in us. The beauty of the waterfall was indescribable being actually down a gorge, bordered by sixty foot bamboo. There is so much water in this country that much of it is pure and drinkable. None of us had a problem drinking from the tap. Waterfalls in Costa Rica are ubiquitous, and easy to get to, many having been taken over by entrepreneurs who charged a small admission.

I was getting sore from all the practicing of postures and knew more than I wanted to know about Chakras. A chiropractor was scheduled this day and he arrived promptly at 1 pm. He introduced himself and told us of his lineage coming from the sports medicine machine of California college sports to a stint in Seattle, before making the decision to relocate to Uvita, Costa Rica. The best decision he said he ever made. The longer I am here the more I tend to agree with him.

He answered many of our questions and explained a curious fact about the spine. That the disc, in the back, between the vertebrae has fluid in it, but is not continually supplied with Synovial fluid, as is the knee when the movement of the knee calls for it. The only thing that keeps the disc healthy and fluid is constant motion, not sitting in one place as we do at our desks. In fact he said that sitting too long, more than four hours a day is as bad for your health as being a regular smoker. He also told us to never do a standing pose with weight on a locked knee, something that is a regular part of the Bikram sequence. I had been doing this for eight years, go figure. The teachers there also told me the Bikram idea of a triangle was actually an extended side angle, and that a triangle was done on straight, but widened legs.

I was pleasantly surprised at his presentation, and he is a regular Yoga practitioner, his wife being a yoga teacher.

Later that afternoon, we again took to the jungle platform to practice our asanas and corrections to them. We were eating nothing but vegetarian meals three times a day, and there was no smoking, drinking or drugs allowed the whole 25 days. All of this was not a problem for me having been sober a while, and having an aversion to drugs American Big Pharma is trying to kill us with, but not before emptying our pockets, as thoroughly as possible, before lowering the body into its' hole. Much of Latin America, I found, rely on herbal medicines that have kept folks healthy for years. My new friend Ray, the Doctor, informed me of how many places below Costa Rica , the USA is, in areas of health care and mortality. Probably why CR was not mentioned as a "Shithole" country.

I had been going to bed by 8 since I got here trying to plan my sleep around the rooster next door and the ever changing numbers of small dogs that barked all night for no apparent reason, but to piss of my Yogi mellow, mind. It is not so much the yoga that is tiring but the sitting on a wooden platform day after day for several hours in the heat. I was used to drinking tons of water from living in Arizona and taking hot yoga, but that didn't mean that this new experience, wasn't tiring. I told my wife that I felt a bit like being in Yoga lockdown, and forced to meditate after trying to escape. But this too shall pass. I hit my twin bed at 8.

----------Even the desire for liberation is a bondage------

This morning I woke earlier and felt more rested because the rooster had a bad night and didn't start crowing until 4:30. We were headed to the Ocean this morning to meditate do some sitting postures, take pictures for their website and frolic in the waves. We walked as a group the 30 minutes to the Ocean passing many dirt roads and out of the way restaurants and boutique hotels no bigger than a three bedroom home. The size of the trees on the way to the ocean seemed to get bigger as we approached. This I sensed was odd. Usually the vegetation dies off when the Ocean is reached, but here the actual rainforest stopped only twenty or thirty feet from the water. Approaching the ocean was so picturesque. I had to catch my breath. Large foamy waves breaking hugely, (trump word) against dark wet volcanic sand. The air over the waves was a mist and the smell of the air was especially fragrant as it is in all of this land covered in bougainvillea and bird of paradise, and wild hydrangea. Our fearless leader who has a body like a gymnast and who also is an excellent meditation leader and practitioner, and masseuse, found a spot for us to sit and meditate.

We formed a circle and began to listen to her gentle voice. I happened to look up and saw that I was seated under a 60 ft coconut tree, displaying several nearly ripened coconuts. I had seen warnings about not parking or sleeping or spending any length of time under them and now I clearly understood why. I had never envisioned my obituary would read "Meditating man killed, reached Samadhi, by falling coconut." I think I would rather be killed by a jealous lover than go out by coconut. That would at least be gossip worthy. I moved back slowly to get away from the possible path of a falling coconut while at the same time keeping an eye on another of our chaperones who was wincing at me for breaking the circle as it was set up. I was not willing to die on principle. I stopped when I thought I was safe, but didn't know if I should warn the woman next to, and now in front of me, who was from Austria, that she too was risking her life under the tree. I reasoned that Austria had far better health care than the U.S., so I said nothing and closed my eyes. Just then a tremendous roar barked through the dense trees along the beach road. It didn't sound like a dog, if it were a dog it would have to be a big one and a baritone. It was a Howler monkey and it continued through her whole meditation. You will never hear anything eerier than a Howler monkey, and it seemed to be not far behind me and I hoped that the noise did not get any louder. Coincidentally the monkey stopped howling, when she stopped the meditation. Maybe the monkey had had enough of the Yogis meditating in his front yard, maybe he was a Yang monkey not into being one with the universe? The photographer then showed up and the women all ran to the water and started planning all kinds of playful, but difficult poses on the sand. Tara, from Holland,and I performed a facing hand connected Dancer pose, then I attempted a headstand, but the waves rushed in washed away the sand and I fell on my ass, which was also captured on disc. The water was warm and the waves beautiful, the view in every direction was spectacular. There were a few surfers scattered about and a few walkers. There seemed to be many squatters who had quickly thrown together shacks along the beach road not 50 ft from the water. I wondered why the government allowed this on such beautiful land. I suppose I'll never know. It was time to walk to the bus that would take us back to Yoga camp for more talk on Chakras, Dukkha, Apana, Pranayama, Mudras, Nadis, Samadhi, and correcting asanas. Things could be worse…I could be stuck in Baltimore, in February. Or trying to explain the eight limbs of yoga. Which are as follows since I failed to get even one correct on my test.

1.Yama…regulation or middle ground.
2.Niyama…observences, training. 3.Asana..posture training…4.Pranayama..breath control. 5. Pratyahara.. withdrawal of senses…6. Dharana…concentration..7. Dhyana…meditation…8. Samadhi…super conscious state. Enlightenment.

---------Forget all you have learned, become a child again—Sri Paramahamsa

Today was the last day of the first full week of our Yoga training. On this day all of us would be pulled aside and interviewed about how we felt about being there, and how we felt overall. I had my concerns about the rooster and the dogs and the heat out on the platform in the afternoon. But I didn't want to seem like "that guy", an old guy complaining, so on my interview I simply said that we could have practiced longer on the beach, and had more beach time. Otherwise all was well. I had meditated regularly at a temple in New York that was next to a firehouse and we would sit through that noise. The goal after all is to accept the outside world as it is and ignore it. I had made friends with a Buddhist monk during his stay in Arizona and I would regularly smuggle in to the temple his favorite food, Big Macs, and not just one, had to be two. So everything has parameters that stretch and yawn, so I let all else be. I did mention the rooster.

After our individual interview sessions we were broken into two's and had to do a skit defining a line in the Bhagavad Gita, Hindu Holy Scripture, so me and Maria from Argentina decided to rap this particular line of scripture.

She danced behind me while I bounced around like Eminem, wording the truth.

" Delusion is you know it's not real, but you want to believe it is.

But let me tell you Yogi friend your suffering increases if you hold onto it.

This too shall pass like a body full of gas, and nothing lasts forever bye bye.

My advice is to take a look in the mirror, take a good look twice.

You'll see the reality of your world, in which you live, is really very nice."

I thought this was not too bad for an old white guy, Maria wrote most of it, and it went over pretty well with our group. Then it was time to hit the platform in the jungle.

We worked through our presentations of our final exam which would include teaching a 60 minute class using 5 major asana groups, inversion, twist, standing, and seated posture, and pranayama (deep breathing). Toward the end of the days training one of our teachers tried to explain the Bondas . when she realized most of us were falling asleep she called it a day and we went through a back to back meditation where we sat against another persons' back and then we stood up, arms still locked, and hugged that person and then we group hugged. This was a lot of hugging for me in one day, not that it's not all good but I was feeling a bit awkward about being too good. My inner child needing to be spanked?

---------------No good deed goes unpunished-------

A week ago while watching the super bowl at the restaurant in town I spied a large cheesecake on the top shelf of their display. I had been thinking about that cheesecake all week and also about the chocolate covered doughnut sprinkled with nuts at the bakery just before the main road. After our vegetarian dinner of some kind of green soup, which was in fact tasty, I thought I would take a walk into town. It didn't take me long and I walked into the restaurant and right to the display case and sure enough the pie was there. Probably not the same one I noticed a week ago but it looked like it. I asked the waiter in my broken Spanish what it was and how much. He told me it was 3800 colonies and that it was Coconut cheesecake. I ordered a piece and sat down. It was about 5 U.S.D.

Just as I sat down to wait for it to be delivered to my table, in walks the owner of the Yoga school and her family. Oh shit, I thought, I don't want to gobble this down, and I don't want her to see me. Karma, I thought. Luckily they ordered to go and were soon out of the restaurant. The cake was brought to me with only a spoon. I summoned the waitress to get me a fork, and I tried to make a fork sign with my fingers. She came back with a knife. I was dying to eat this thing and had to suffer the pain of attachment. I shook my head and having no other good choices she finally brought me a fork. I tried not to eat too fast. My first non- veggie food in a week. I tried the Buddhist, thirty chews per bite, routine but couldn't stick to it. I walked back to the camp after enjoying the tasty cake. Past the bakery that I would visit in the morning. It was a long week," I'm too old for this," I sometimes thought ,but many people at my age can't even leave the house without pain, I should be thankful, even if I have to sneak cake. This whole thing was going to be a bucket list adventure for real. Tomorrow I will head for Jaco the party town up the road, the surfing Mecca, with a casino and many tourists and where prostitution is legal, actually it is in the whole country. Not that I would be into that, in keeping to my training, but to see the action would be let's say, enlightening?

-----You need not fight a habit, just don't give it an opportunity to repeat itself—

Saturday morning and 9 am, I walked out of our ashram toward the bus depot on my way to Jaco and a 2 hour bus trip. The bus depot was nearby and when I got there I was informed that there was not a bus to Jaco, but a direct bus to San

Jose, but that I could get off on hwy 34, and take a cab in. So I boarded the bus after giving the driver my money and checking twice with him that he would let me off, he kept smiling and shaking his head " Si,Si". The beautiful thing about Costa Rica is that people in the service industry will go out of their way to make things easier for you, unlike in the US where seemingly every extra nicety one asks for takes an act of Congress, when they are not on vacation. Or they will give you 15 different reasons why you can't be accommodated. The ride didn't seem like 2 hours and as promised he dropped me off on the side of the highway, where there were an abundance of cabs willing to take me to town for 1000 colonies, about 2 USD. It was not quite a mile and I wasn't going to walk it. I was resting over the weekend, recharging the beast. Detoxing the rooster.

I found my hotel the Cadillac Rock right next to the Beatle bar, which seemed crowded with ex-pats. I later found out why. I had walked the entire length of the strip twice, had already bought myself a couple of cooler shirts not counting on the humidity here, and a couple pairs of shorts. I decided after a short nap to walk the strip again since it was now 7 o'clock and things may be picking up. As I walked nearing the end of the strip a voice in my head said, "Why don't you cross the street and see what's over there?" Without so much as a second thought, I did. I stepped on the curb glanced at a guy carrying a Yoga mat and he yelled out, "Hey Al that you?" It was my Yin Yoga teacher who taught teacher training a month earlier in Phoenix. At that time I felt a connection with him and took him to lunch during our training."Oh my God, Yoga James!" It was Yoga James (his website name) and his female companion KB. Almost bumping into me. We hugged and laughed and chuckled at the Karma of all this. I knew he was doing yoga sessions at the Envision Festival, end of February, but didn't think he would be in the country this soon. They were in the process of trying to find an Air BnB and I stopped them. "I have two beds in my room why don't you take one. If you don't mind sleeping with me." "Not at all," they seemed to say in unison. So I walked back to the hotel while they grabbed a bite to eat and I laid down and waited for them. I was sleeping by the time they came in but the next morning we talked for hours about The Eight Limbs of Yoga and Nadis, and Chakras, and the necessity in some circles of transcending the mind to get deeper into Yoga. We finally agreed to leave the mind alone, it was doing the best it could from where it came. Breakfast was delicious on the strip and I learned that the Beatles bar next door to my hotel was quite the pick up place for the ex-pats to employ the local ladies of the night. I had heard that prostitution was legal here but had no idea I'd be so close, and be in bed at 8 pm to boot. I also noticed when I checked in, a full scale cardboard cutout of The Beatles performing on my hotel porch. I got up at six, Sunday morning, while the two of them slept, and practiced my asana sequence on the beach and then spent almost an hour playing in the warm ocean with the sun coming up over the mountains. It was magical. After we had chatted and had breakfast it was time for me to use my limited Spanish to get my butt back to Yoga camp by evening. Actually getting around Costa Rica is not that hard. The main highway 34 comes straight from San Jose and goes along the coast. Stopping at the three or 4 of the most major towns. The local busses run more often and will get you where you want quicker in most cases. My trip was an example. The bus coming from San Jose on Rt. 34 went as far as Uvita (the last stop) only twice on Sunday, 9 am and passing through Jaco at 4 to reach Uvita by 6. However there was a local bus out of Jaco at 12:30 to Quespos, with a transfer to Uvita at 2:30. So that's what I did. The local from Quespos stopped at every little hamlet, but it was after all the local. In any event I was home by 4pm, in time to have dinner with Tara one of the teacher assistants, herself a Bikram student, from Holland. When I got back my bed was changed and room cleaned up a bit. I was not as tired as I thought I would be the next day. The main teacher always took us through a fairly good workout of astanga and vinyassa, that lasted about ninety minutes and then we spent the rest of the morning breaking down each asana and learning modifications to those poses for students who were simply not physically able to do the full expression. After lunch we broke into groups of two, three, or four, to practice teach a sequence that we made up that had to include, pranayama breathing, backbends, sun salute, inversions, sitting postures, spine twist, standing warm-up postures and a 10 minute meditation. This morning we were joined by another howler monkey who apparently got bored after a couple of sequences and stopped howling.

We had been doing a lot of one on one and getting quite close and learning a lot about each other. I had not been to such a touchy feely affair in quite some time save the AA campout in Sedona in October, that proved to be liberating for me.

I found out one of the women was on the scene in Stockholm when a terrorist blew up a truck severing her friend's leg. She stayed with her friend until paramedics arrived but still suffers from PTSD, can you blame her. I told her about tapping and that she should look into that . It is said that you can learn more about a person in an hour of play, than in a year of relationship. I now believe that having been immersed in sudden outbursts of group hugs, free style spontaneous dance, defense breakdown staring and touching, all to break down the ego and bring about bonding.

--- Ignorance, egoism, attachment, hatred and clinging to bodily life, are the five obstacles to Samadhi. ----

Finally I was seeing the light at the end of the tunnel. The beautiful young women among us with the very fit bodies seemed to be tiring out before the end of our ten hour days, and I was still hanging in. Exhausted, but hanging in. I was dutifully taking my amino acid powder mixed with Maca and it seemed to be giving me the extra energy it always had. Now the teachers were starting to notice and I believe, were planning more indoor activities for us and book work.

Today we listened to Lee the school's oldest student, I was the second oldest. He hadn't started yoga until age 65 when he retired but he went after it with a vengeance, God bless him, and was now teaching chair yoga to vets and seniors in Arkansas. He is in great shape and imparted many useful asanas in his afternoon talk and singing bowl meditation. This was our 7th day of class and technically hump day and I was relieved. I walked down the street to pick up my laundry , two dollars to have a few shorts and tops washed and I walked another block to the market for a snickers before going back to the Yoga studio for more vegetarian food. Lunch as it was called, Most of it was palatable but indistinguishable.

Everyone on staff here, the leader and owner who had practiced in India earning a 300 hour certificate, on top of her 200 hour certificate, and the other 5 teacher assistants were very helpful and friendly, and made the place feel like home. Mara who ran the dormitory and kitchen is a sweetheart too as is her husband Julio.

We had spent countless hours the past few days learning a breathing technique called Nadi Suddhi, where one presses the left nostril breathes in through the right, and then reverses this and alternates breathing with a variety of different nostril combinations. I asked the (soon to be) doctor in our group if there wasn't an area behind the nose where all the air combines anyway and goes down the trachea. He appeared to know where I was going with this and laughed and nodded yes there is. I couldn't see myself, how alternate use of the nostrils made any difference at all. It's not like the left nostril only supplied the left lung? "You're gonna make a good doctor." I chuckled. Go with the flow, I kept telling myself. Don't rock the boat, be teachable, not a know- it-all. And so that conversation will go with me to the grave.

Time was starting to pass quicker now but the yoga in the morning was no easier. I was not using modifications but the sequences were still difficult. We practiced our 5 minute Pranayama, breathing sequence, again today along with our ten minute guided meditation, also required, on the platform late this afternoon. As a group we were hanging in there and I had the sense that this event would be a life long memory and generate some life long friends, I felt myself going from petrified, to skeptical to happy, and the patient staff had a lot to do with it. It's almost eight so I'm going to bed now to beat the rooster.

-------There is no value in digging shallow wells in a hundred places. Decide on one place and dig deep.--------

Today is Valentines day and we meandered along the narrow path over a stream to the platform for morning yoga. I had gotten a decent night's sleep beating the rooster who didn't start crowing until 3:47 am but continued till at least 9. I was toying with the idea of buying the rooster from this neighbor, how much could a rooster cost?, and donating it to the church down the road. Then I decided not to rock the boat and simply turn it over, to a Higher Power. We enjoyed a rather slow paced gentle 90 minute workout and then paired up for Thai massage training.

Maria from Argentina happened to be next to me and we paired off. We were instructed on several different massage techniques including holding on to each other while we did backbends and various other holding massages and the final one had us use our hands and knees to go up the back of the legs including the butt and back and neck. It couldn't have been a more pleasant morning. Then at the end the teacher had us dance around like crazy and everyone just went wild. Fun things like this are good I think did break the stress of ten hour days, in this humidity. We gathered in the concrete hall before lunch for headstand, handstand and uplift asanas. Then we took a hike about a half mile to the river to talk about Teacher ethics, and take a swim. Just before the river we hiked through a bamboo forest with bamboo over 90 ft high and nearly a foot thick. It was an amazing site. The river was beautiful and colder than the ocean but crystal clear. The thousands of little tadpoles in the water and miniature frogs, that they would soon become were overlooked by us, since they seemed to be doing no harm, we were invading their space. At the end of the day we performed another touchy feely exercise where we picked a partner and had to stare for 5 minutes into one of their eyes without any emotion or laughter. Me and the British woman next to me teamed up and began staring at each other. She was older than the rest of the girls, and married and settled. This exercise was more uncomfortable than I had anticipated. The last time I tried something like this it was when I was high and part of a mating ritual I'm sure. I told her that, when it was finally over, and she laughed and said she was thinking the same thing. We both tried not to laugh or snicker and finally calmed down enough to do this exercise.

Tomorrow I get to wear my snake boots because after yoga we are going to gather medicinal plants from the property. I had seen, which I never should have, a Netflix film on the 50 deadliest creatures in Central America. One of the deadliest snakes, the Fer de Lance, or two step snake lived here. I noticed however, that the snake hunters who gathered for anti-venom were wearing knee high rubber boots. I went to Cal ranch cowboy store before I left and to my surprise found a pair my size for 30 bucks. These were, of course, used to clean out horse stalls, but they looked like snake boots to me, so I bought them and brought them along. If I don't use them by the time I leave, I am gifting them to Julio of our casa. They have buckles in front like the ones I had in third grade.

------   Enlightenment: When one is perfectly content, with everything being imperfect------

This morning we opened our practice on the platform with an entire session on Shavasana, the most popular pose, or "corpse pose." To continue to lie down with my eyes closed was a blessing. The hour and a half went by quickly. My partner this day was a young woman from Philadelphia who happened to be a masseuse. Lucky me, I tried to return the favor when it was her turn in Shavasana, but she knew her stuff better than I, but we both got a good massage.

We then were scheduled to walk the property with Nestor a Florida transplant who was into cultivating naturally growing plants for production. This he had done in Florida. His tour was interesting, showing us what lemon grass looked like and its' medicinal purposes as well as a host of other plants that needed boiling before consuming or whether they could be eaten raw. He mentioned that there are dozens of varieties of banana plants even in Costa Rica. He pointed out bird of paradise and their version of wandering jew. This is an incredibly luscious country due to its position on the globe, seven degrees from the equator, and because of the rainfall, which exceeds 10 inches per month for several months beginning in June. In fact most travel guides advise not to visit during the months of heavy rainfall due to road washouts and other dangerous conditions due to flooding.

We went over the business end of Yoga after lunch and argued about what kind of salary a yoga teacher could make. We were shown statistics that indicate the lifestyle has grown 400% since 2010.

With the largest growth in Japan. However at 35 dollars a class no one becomes a teacher for the money but for the satisfaction in helping others to a better life.

At the end of the day we participated in a New Moon ceremony, and used a Death arrow where we chose a stick and filled it with thoughts of what we wanted to get rid of for the coming year, those things that no longer served us. We stood around the fire turned to the west to thank Father Sky for his protection and then to the north to thank Mother Earth, then south and east to thank other mothers and fathers. Next in groups of four we threw our sticks into the fire. The biggest Death arrow was passed around and each of us took it and prayed separately. Then the youngest, Siddhara from UK, and I the oldest, walked this arrow to the fire and threw it in. We sang and chanted until that arrow had completely burned. I felt like the old man on Survivor, but I wasn't yet being voted off, I was being quiet and cooperating and accepting all the woo, woo as fact even though the Indian Gurus who come up with this stuff can't agree on its' meaning or value to yoga or to samadhi. This little ceremony was however pagan in nature and commonly done in Iceland. Who knew? I decided and was encouraged to take what I could use and leave the rest, as is true for all religions. Why?" Because in experiencing God, you transcend the mind, God cannot be understood by the mind, because mind is matter, and matter cannot possibly understand something more subtle than matter." The truth is we don't know the face of God, only the energy that does God's work and we observe the results in our lives. Once we accept our humanity and stop competing with God for a place at his chair, and accept our brokenness, we are liberated and able to surrender, and Samadhi becomes possible.

I went through my asana sequence with one of the teachers before our burning ceremony, only to find out that many of my postures didn't flow properly and required too much shifting of the feet. This was depressing since the final presentation of our 60 minute class to the rest of the class started Monday, two days from now. I wanted to know it as well as possible without stammering and being stuck not knowing how to talk a student into or out of a posture, so my weekend is going to be spent on the beach recording my voice and trying to understand my sequence. Life could be worse, in fact it became so the following day

After a particularly difficult Astanga yoga morning warm-up on the platform we were advised that we were going to an organic self-supporting farm in the mountains, that was owned by an American University and run by a couple of professors. Carlos the manager spoke little English but just enough to throw the women in the group into a "tell me more" head spin. His abundant black hair was rolled on top of his head and his gracious searching accent, was contagious. He showed us how he sharpened his Machete, and that the machete was always with him and an overall necessity in Costa Rica. That was the first thing out of his mouth, how sharp his machete was. This worried me a little and I hoped he never had to use it except to open pipas, or coconuts.

The farm was just beautiful with pineapples growing in planted rows. I learned that they don't grow on trees. Don't know why I thought they did? We were hiking to the waterfall about 3,000 feet below us at a 30% grade. This was the time I needed my snake boots but had left them back favoring my Merrell hikers. It took us a while to get to the waterfall and we watched as Carlos and his brother hacked some bushes that had fallen on our path. "Carlos please tell me there is a shorter way back ?" I moaned. "Yes the other way." Was all he said in broken English. I was, however relieved that there was another way. I asked him earlier if they ever see any of my friends the fer de lance snake. He said that they do but only occasionally, because they usually come out at night or dusk. He said if he sees one he usually tries to kill it because it may kill someone else. They used to call this snake the two stepper. Referring to how many steps one could take after being bitten before hitting the ground a dead man. I was relieved when he told me that no, you would have about four hours to get the anti-venom before dying. I was pretty sure we were four hours from a Vet, since they carry the anti-venom. All this was going through my mind as I stumbled down the hiking trail, to the waterfall. Alas after it was over and we swam in the crystal clear water, Carlos opened coconuts for all of us and the milk was refreshing, as was the meat inside. Upon arriving back at our Yoga house I learned that my presentation was to be the last one on the last morning, Friday that we were to graduate and leave. Mine was 6 am. At least I would be fresh, I thought, and would be able to listen to the others ahead of time. I was concerned that I did not have enough asanas (postures) for 60 minutes, and that my calling them out, knowing when to call for an inhale or exhale would be off point. I added more sitting postures and few standing postures, and a few from Pilates that would be a little surprise, but what the hey, the teacher used a few Pilates mat poses, in her presentation why couldn't I? My roommate Joel later used a Lou Ferrigno hulk flexing pose in his presentation. Never saw that before, probably never will again lol.

I practiced my sequence with Maria from Argentina, she had such a direct controlling sense of humor and for some reason I like that. Telling me "No not like that like these." I like the way she says "speen " your ankles, instead of spin. I told her what spin meant, when she asked me to roll my ankles. Same thing I supposed?

-----The moment you have surrendered, and resigned, is the moment you have transcended your own ego----

For some reading this book, and having a Yoga retreat in Costa Rica on their bucket list, a few thoughts on my experience, to pass on. If you are over 35, I would go with a friend since the majority of students in all teacher trainings outside of India, are in their twenty's. Going with a friend will make it more fun. The kids here try to include me in trips and outings but I feel somewhat like a fifth wheel. Also don't pick a Yoga school based on price. I did that and got what I paid for. A rooster and 3 vegetarian meals a day. However the staff is great and checked in on how everyone was feeling once a week. Get your own room with air conditioning, a guarantee of a quiet sleep, save the howler monkeys, and a reasonably well rounded choice of local food. Ask about a refund if in the first day or so the experience is not what you expected, most will agree to that and then you have only paid for airfare. You can hang around and make a vacation out of it. If possible attend an Adult training, some schools offer this, where everyone has to be over 35 or 40 years old. Be aware of the humidity in Central America. I got a good Yoga education from a wonderful staff, and I appreciate that but knowing what I do now, I would have tried to tie up the loose ends for myself by choosing to be more comfortable, at a price, of course. This is a magical country, make no mistake, the people here are wonderful and the cooperation one feels is contagious. There is no fear of walking the streets here like in the U.S., even at night, and no us versus them mentality. In time the U.S.A. ego will destroy itself, and join the ranks of third world countries. I can easily see why there are so many ex-pats here from all over the globe. You will love it here especially not getting Fox News, and everywhere you look is like a post card from Survivor the show.

Already the Millennials in my class, from other countries in Europe and South America, wonder why the U.S. is so unkind to its' citizens. I shrug since I don't have an answer, I let my embarrassment speak for itself. Yesterday morning we had a Disney Yoga class where we played Disney songs and danced around the platform after class, Today we sat in a circle with another person in front of us and gave that person a backrub. These are things I would get to do nowhere else, and are good for me to let go and surrender to the moment. Then we did lion's breath and let our tongues hang out on our exhale making loud roaring sounds.

For who am I really, who is anyone? I was born with a body and a skeleton of a personality that is constantly, even at my age morphing. I am a Yogi, I am a father, I am a drummer, I am bisexual, I am a singer, I am a Democrat, and on and on, but just as I am all these things I am not one of them. I realized not long ago that I don't have to make choices in my live to give up any part of who I am because that doesn't fit into some one's idea of a role, male or female. As Shakespeare said "We are all actors on a stage." And we play certain roles at certain times either because that is required of us or because we want to and it's fun. A cop doesn't behave at home with his family the way he does on the job. And we all have certain roles we play either consciously or unconsciously, to get what we want , or to be left alone. The only true identity any of us have is that we are children of God, since like in any family we are all different and complex and have our own journey. That's ok. This three week training has forced me to lighten up, when I never realized how uptight I was in the first place. Most of the fun had gone from my life, and it was my own fault for not looking for it. According to Patanjali the causes of bondage and liberation are in our own minds. If we think we are bound we are bound. If we think we are liberated we are liberated. Because you think you are living you are living. If you applied you mind to the thought that you are dying you would die. It is only when we transcend the mind that we are free from all these troubles. We should realize that we are completely different from the mind. We are eternally free, never bound.

------If you are going to be selfish, be selfish in maintaining your own peace of mind------

Later in the day, after I had already taken three classes, we were going to tackle arm balance postures. A couple of the teachers were of Astanga training where those kinds of postures are common. For the average Yoga practitioner, they are exceedingly difficult but then some poses are just balancing tricks. Toward the end of our session someone asked how to do a tripod headstand. I had done that posture at the Arizona Regional's in 2014 and ended up in first place. The teacher had seen me do it earlier and said "Alan can do that why don't you do it for us Alan?" So I did. I came into a crow asana where I balance on my inner arms, then tip forward onto my head and use my core to bring my legs into a headstand. Then I spread my legs wide brought them back together, went into Garrasana (eagle) feet wrapping my calves around each other, came out of that into an uplift and plopped down . The others thought that was pretty cool, and I thanked them, knowing I was a one trick pony, that's all I can do of that variety asana. Most of them thought I was at least ten years younger than I am. Maria, from Argentina asked me that this morning after the headstand was posted on our What's Up group. I told her 65, but I'm 67, and she said she thought I was 55. But I know that I've worked hard to maintain my health and it's not just about looks, I want to be able to travel and keep up with the younger folks and get up every morning NOT in pain and not have to feed the Vampire drug companies who really want us dead or broke. And the only way I know to accomplish that is to take care of myself by myself and watch what I put in my mouth, and exercise.

As we were winding up the afternoon on the platform a group of White faced Capuchin monkeys started through the treetops in front of our platform and came down for a drink in the stream that ran by the platform. A few of the younger monkeys watched us critically from their perch, sometimes hanging by only their tail while picking out just the right leaf to snack on while watching us struggle with something so easy for these yoga masters. There seemed to be a scattering and yelping among the monkey tribe and suddenly the largest among them worked its way down from his perch and stood not more than ten feet from Nikki with two K's, and started hissing and showing its teeth, seeming to be quite agitated. The teacher grabbed her water bottle and ran toward the angry monkey, scaring it back up into the tree. We all stopped what we were doing, as surprised as the teacher was that one would be so aggressive. We had seen this troupe come by before and we never had any problem with them except that for a few moments the second day, they threw water apples at us from the top of the tree in our courtyard. They are cute but are certainly not pets and know full well how to unzip a backpack with food inside. We never left food out in the kitchen since it was open to the outside with no windows, only the bedrooms had windows. We called the big one Oscar and assumed he was the alpha male.

------Ignorance is regarding the impermanent as permanent, the impure as pure, the painful as pleasant, and the non-self as the self.---------

Today is Wednesday and we have one more day of class. Tomorrow 3 of my friends give their classes so it will be another three yoga session, day for me. Friday morning there is just my class and graduation and we are done at noon. Some of the girls are going to the Envision Festival which is a big deal here with plenty of music and Hippie wear. I even bought a top for Nikki with two K's since she was going to the festival and had nothing cool to wear. It had fringe on it and looked great on her, as anything would really. I was able to get in as a volunteer but could not work out a schedule to work that didn't interfere with my returning flight, so I had to cancel. Maria and the girls here want to see Xavier Rudd, who I had never heard of, but they played me some of his songs and he sounds like a new version of John Mayer or John Sebastian, but I liked his tunes. I told Maria I was writing a book about my trip here. Previously she said, " You chould write a book aboud yer sperience here to give hope to older peoples, and cho them bout you." I loved to hear her accent, It was so hot, and as you know from reading this, so was she. Her accent kind of reminded me of a female Ricky Riccardo, from the Lucy Show. She shared that she was 34 and had had a boyfriend that she had to leave because of his drinking, but she seems content to travel through Central America, not looking to settle down, or take just any job. I always envied folks like that since I always panicked during my lifetime, and took a job to keep food on the table even if it was something I didn't care for. Kids are different today and I applaud that. Know yourself, be alone, there are plenty of single people to do stuff with. I guess I was always co-dependent from not getting enough hugs or believing I might starve to death.

This evening class involved couples yoga and acro-yoga and because I came late to the platform and everyone else had paired up, I was paired with Amber one of the teachers. To describe her would not do her justice. At about 5 ft tall with long brown hair and massive thighs and a cute butt and a great knowledge of Yoga and meditation she could easily be on the cover of any sports or girlie magazine. A perfectly chiseled face with a gorgeous smile, cute turned up nose and twinkling eyes. But enough about her. We were going to demonstrate couples yoga. In front of the class I was seated back to back with her, and after following her directions, somehow found myself with my head in her lap and hers in mine, and I'm not really sure where my feet and legs were. After not having much human contact for the last three weeks my massage by her this evening after class, was going to be difficult to bear.

Then we demonstrated other postures where we ended up holding each other up by leaning into each other, hands to hands, She told me to get closer and kiss noses, so I kissed her nose. That was not what she meant. It was what I had hoped I heard, but not what she meant. She meant to touch noses, like Eskimos, but hey I'm from Arizona where there are no Eskimos. We did a back to back Warrior 2, both sides and then came the acro-yoga. She had me balancing on her feet with my hands behind my back doing a forward fold over her feet and other such things. I actually had my arms out like an airplane balancing only on her feet. By the time we were done, after we had chanted 108 times, she gave me a massage that was wonderful but brutal. I asked her if she got hit on by tourists who ever asked her about happy endings, since she was so beautiful. All she said was "No". and plopped me on her table like a rag doll. She tore into my back like a Roto-tiller but it's what I needed, whether or not my question deserved punishment. Earlier in the day the owner asked us to give her school good reviews on line, and I saw no reason not to. It wasn't their fault that there was a rooster nearby, although in a third world country you would think someone would have a gun handy, it would have made a tasty meal.

-----Understanding of truth is totally different from knowledge gained from study of scripture ------ Similarly, standing in a garage, does not make you a car.----

I was starting to become Namastayed out. I was beginning to tire of all the circles and mantras and chakras and vegetarian food. I tip toed to the bakery last evening when I went to the bank, and brought back a triangle shaped cream filled croissant with chocolate and nuts on top. I snuck it into my room and opened it the minute I awoke. Yes there were ants in the box, but they were small, and I was able to brush them off and devour it, not without sharing a bit with my roomy. He is a quirky kid from Clearwater Florida, with a keen brain and a lot of needy energy. He kind of reminded me of me back at his age, anything for a laugh or to get noticed. He may have been devoid of hugs as a child like I was. We are all broken aren't we? That's why we are here. To try and heal the brokenness inside us.

With that thought in mind, I talked to the wife today about her arthritis pain and the problem that presents for her. We talked about diet and stress and such, and she mentioned a curious question being asked by our friends who are aware of what I'm doing in Costa Rica. "What does he plan to do with that?"(teaching certificate). This kind of thinking, unfortunately is symptomatic of the me generation who are now Seniors and plan on retiring to a life of drinking, golf, and pickleball. What about giving back to the community and the World? What about mentoring some young people? What about learning new things from exposure to young people? It is said that he who stops growing dies. It is a shame that older folks don't think they have anything to offer the next generation and vice versa. We shut our minds as we grow older thinking we know everything and that there is no more to learn. Mano went to his masters' house for tea eager to tell him everything he had learned on his visit to the temple. He sat down and Tyko the Master poured him his tea as Mano went on about his newly gained knowledge. Tyko allowed the tea to spill over the cup burning Mano."Ouch Master why didn't you stop pouring?" he screamed " Because your mind is like that cup, so full that nothing else will fit, and you hear no one but yourself." The thought that I might enjoy teaching other folks yoga apparently escaped their conscious mind. Probably knowing that teaching is a lot of work for little money, made no sense for them. Had I been going to teacher training for Financial Planning they wouldn't have said a word. To so many people including those in political power, money and power have become their God, and they worship at the alter of consumerism and ego, at their own peril.

The bad news this morning is that my 1962 Rolling Stones flip flops broke on my way out to the Yoga platform. Julio who runs this place, to whom I gave my snake boots, offered to take them to a shoe repairer on his dime. I so hope it works. This is our last full day here, after my presentation at 6 am there is breakfast and graduation ceremony. Then I will be a full fledged 200 hour RYT.. Registered Yoga Teacher.

My yoga mate Michelle from the U.K. just gave her class and the white faced monkeys soon arrived most of us were watching them climb and swing from vine to tree eating the leaves but seeming to be particular in what leaves they wanted from the same tree. It was quite a treat seeing these things make absolute fools of us with their acrobatics and swinging effortlessly through the jungle, many times using only their tales to wrap around a vine and pick out just the right leaf to eat, while hanging upside down. These are the true Yogis. Perhaps they have adopted the Yoga platform as their play place and we were using it? We will never know, the most exciting class I ever took, but this time no advancing angry Oscar.

-------People soon forget what you say..and sooner forget what you do..But no one will forget the way you made them feel.----------

Today our last day, my teaching day, and graduation. Last night I had to bow out of yet another set of astanga practice, after doing three other yoga classes to support my mates. I was beginning to feel a bit Yoga'd out .I had been Namastaed to death, Chakra'd into submission and generally a good boy. I had only complained about the rooster to the owner in our weekly chats and only mentioned that I would like more beans for lunch. After all we were in a Latino country and I had grown accustomed to beans and rice from Living in another Latino country, Arizona. I did start to see beans appearing for lunch and they were quite tasty. However there were classes after lunch and this gave new meaning to the "Wind release pose."

The rooster is still at large with a bounty on it's head since the neighbor insists that it is not his.

Three of us went out for dinner last night to avoid yet another vegetarian meal. We had a favorite spot a few doors down from the Yoga camp. My roommate, and one of the teaching assistants and myself, ordered Chili cheese fries, chicken wings, Buffalo style, and fries covered with vegetables and cheese.

We were in heaven, it took us a few hours, to consume the huge servings offered. It started raining heavily as we were finishing and at first I didn't know whether I should run or walk back. As I darted out into the heavy rain I immediately slowed down to enjoy the warm thick rain. After all it probably rains here in an afternoon as much as it does in a year in Phoenix. I walked slowly back to our rooms leaving my two dinner partners to walk behind, since they were having some kind of affair and I wanted to give them space to put together their puzzle, and because they were stoned and I was not. I wanted to keep a clear head for my class at 6 am, in the jungle. It was fun getting completely drenched by rain, warm rain. I had not purposely done that since I was very young.

As I prepared for bed I realized that I should not have ordered the chicken wings. These were some of the best tasting wings I had ever had but the hot sauce was just that, HOT sauce. To be kept up all night was the last thing I wanted to happen, but it nearly did. I managed to get enough sleep and woke up at five without my alarm in time to shower and get my things for the walk to the platform. I had never gone through the jungle this early in the morning when it was still dark and some of the women mentioned the feeling of being watched out by the platform. Apparently there are tree cats almost as big as a jaguar or leopard common to this area, but never the less powerful. I also worried about snakes, having given my snake boots to Julio. I had torn my 1962 Rolling Stones flip flops yesterday and was counting on Julio to have them repaired, since I gave him my boots. I thought that if a cat came after me I would throw my yoga mat on it and wrestle around on top of it until it ran away. This kind of thinking only happens in the mind of someone who watches too many Superhero movies or re-runs of Baywatch. I simply resigned myself to the fact that if I didn't make it to the platform, I would be torn to shreds and dragged up into a tree, as a meal for the cat for a couple of weeks, so I wouldn't have died in vain. None of that happened as I finally reached the platform only to find two other Yogi's already there. I breathed deeply and started to set up for my class. I had Buddhist monks chanting, ready on my phone and I began to light incense and stick them into the large beams on the platform. The entire class would be there as well as the grading teacher. Since I was last to teach, no one had a reason not to be there.

Promptly at six I greeted the class cheerfully. "Good morning ladies and gentlemen and those of you who still aren't sure." Welcome to Jungle Yoga. That usually got a laugh and is, of course, the opening line in Cabaret. Not the jungle part. My standing series consisted of about 7 asanas including standing stretching, forward folds, Warrior 3, Garassana, Eagle pose, a Bikram on the toes chair, and a traditional chair. I lead them through a series of Warrior one, Warrior two, reverse warrior, Extended side angle and modified side angle, as well as half lift and triangle, with a Vinyasana, before doing the right side, another before the left side and one last one at the end of the set. This the teacher said she liked very much because of the way it flowed. I had planned it to flow but not for any other reason than that I'm lazy and figured that while one is standing you might as well get all the standing postures out of the way and not continue to be popping up and down. Maybe I'll be the inventor of Lazy Yoga that is more like a dance flow than like being at a gym. I got the class on the floor with about fifteen minutes to go and I still had the sitting series and a few prostate postures before Shavasana.

I went a little longer than my allotted 60 minutes simply because there was nothing else planned, but I noticed some of the students looking at their watches. I ignored this and ended

10 minutes later than I should have and set them into Shavasana. I led them through a scenario where their bodies felt like concrete and were being dropped in a large pan of thick fudge. They could feel the warmth and sunk only a little at a time while the warm fudge enveloped their bodies.

I was actually making myself hungry since MY stomach was still churning somewhat from the chicken wings. I stopped the fudge routine and read them something inspirational from "Course on Miracles" " Our deepest fear is not that we are inadequate. It is that we are powerful beyond measure."........

I brought them back to their bodies and out of the fudge and into a sitting meditation posture and guided them into one of my favorite meditations, drawing a triangle from the third eye to each finger until each finger was tingling and the third eye was feeling pressure. The teacher said she loved that personally and felt energy lights pulsing back and forth in her brain. I quoted Mark Twain who said that 98% of everything he worried about never happened. I threw in a little Maya Angelou, "People will forget what you've said, and sooner forget what you've done. But no one will forget the way you made them feel." Then I spoke a bit about the problem of feeling that we are not doing enough in this world and when we feel small always to remember that, "You may be one person in the World, but you may be the World to one person." The class said they enjoyed what I put together and my teacher review was quite good. I was relieved and was ready to go back to the compound. Alas, there was more fun in store. We formed two lines on the platform and grabbed a partner and danced in between the two lines and then the next couple did the same. But wait! There's more.

It was time for heart-breath work while we waited for time to pass until ten o'clock graduation time. We were asked to pair off, and my lovely Maria from Argentina was next to me so it made sense, to nod toward her, she nodded and we paired up. We were to sit facing each other knees to knees, ok been there done that. Next I had to put my hand on her heart which ended up with my thumb also between her breasts and she did the same to me. Next up feeling her breath and adjusting mine to hers,in unison, while staring into her gorgeous dark brown eyes framed by flourishes of reddish brown hair. "Lord thunder and Jesus!" I thought. I had not had sex for over 30 days nor had I masturbated, and here I sit with my hand on the chest of the lovely Maria. I could feel the unease as my brain tried to find a place for this in the now spinning rolodex in my mind. The last time I was in this position I was stoned, preparing for sex, or just stoned, and it was four decades ago. I smiled as she smiled and dared not break the furtive stare we both shared. I felt like the cartoon character with steam coming out of his ears and the word, TILT gleaming from both eyes. I just didn't know where to go or what to do with this so I sat and stared and smiled, until it was over. We did achieve a common breath cycle.

Did things get easier? No. We were asked to find a different partner and I noticed that Nikki, with two K's, was nearby and alone. I definitely had a crush on her too so I asked her to be my partner, and she said ok. Nikki is tall perfectly proportioned has deadly piercing blue eyes and a little baby girl voice that makes you want to grab a fork and help her eat her food. She has copious dark brown curls, stabs you with those eyes while she actually listens to you, and is, well, perfect. This time we were to sit back to back, interlace arms and hold hands while we sat feeling our breath from that direction, back against back, and again instructed to coordinate our breathing. My mind started wandering because I was so tired from the lack of sleep indigestion brings,I began seeing us walking down the aisle, Maria as our bridesmaid, even though she is twenty something and I old enough to be her grandfather. At least Maria is 34 and I still could be her father. I envisioned myself coming up behind her at the coffee machine in my kitchen. She wearing only black lace boy shorts and me, well, nothing, and softly putting my hands on her hips. It took me so long to get that far in my mind that the exercise was soon over, but not before our breath became one. It was no easier now for me to not think sexually about these lovely women, than it was when I first arrived. The difference however, is that I didn't act on it and get grabby or assume things that weren't said or intimated, but only figments of my "bad neighborhood" mind. The hope here was that we had changed from the first day we arrived. Closer to Samadhi?

Now it was time for our actual graduation. We were all asked to wear white and we did. We gathered around the fire that Julio had been trying to start, but couldn't because of the heavy rain the night before. I came off the platform to help him and remembered I had put my final essay in my pocket. I took it out and asked him if some paper would help start the fire, and he gladly took it and smiled. My essay did the trick and the fire ignited enough so that all of us could throw in some symbolic leaves and our old string that was put around our wrists when we first arrived, since we now had new string, symbolizing that we were in fact new people now with all that we had been through. I got that, and did remove the old string, partly because I had now the same color new string and I'm not a big fan of too much string around my wrist. String leads to catching on doors that slam on my heel, usually when I had a load of groceries.

We danced a couple of circles around the fire and sang a couple of songs while a few folks chanted a blessing, in Icelandic because Ziggie was the singer and a good one, and also a medium to the Gods, I told her. Now it was time to hit the platform.

We formed a circle and in the center was a large sheet with the chakras and their colors displayed on it. When your name was called the person next to you walked you to the next person, because you were supposed to close your eyes, and so on until you got back to from whence you came. Each successive person who moved you along had to whisper in your ear something inspirational or motivational, or just tell them how much you enjoyed meeting them. Then that last person would escort you to the center and lay you down on your back, on the chakra sheet. The rest of us would walk forward and put hands on the person lying down and chant one long, loud OM. Then your graduation certificate and a Yoga school t-shirt was placed on your chest, and you were invited to exchange it if it didn't fit, or if you wanted another color. Mine fit and was white so I kept it.

I had a little more intimate of a message for Maria and Nikki, with 2 k's, but said some really nice things to the rest of the group simply because all of them were wonderful soul searching individuals, on a journey to improve their contact with the great Universal Spirit, Higher Power, or God. I was humbled to be among them.

I have always had this haunting feeling when around religious types, Yogis, Reiki practitioners, and Chiropractors, that they somehow sense me as a spiritual fraud or "wanna be" and I can't quite put my finger on it. Is that my fault for not being serious enough, or is it their problem, expecting everyone to be as serious and committed as they. I believe I am very spiritual and I weep a lot when involved in soul searching, inner spirit, rituals and traditions. However there is this little person who looks like Richard Prior, or Dave Chappell, sitting on my shoulder whispering in my ear. " You ain't gonna fall for that shit now are you? Who made this stuff up? You aren't gonna drink this kool- aid are you?" I realize that I'm a skeptic and I've been wrong many times with my "contempt prior to investigation", attitude. I was wrong about Chiropractics, and Reiki, meditation, prayer, acupuncture, that all people at the top of "trickle down" economics were kind enough to trickle down, not on, and the Chicago Cubs. So I stand distant at the depth of these ceremonies, thinking that they exist only to pacify our frail egos and our human preoccupation on "living forever." Together with our collective co-dependence, and desire for a functional family, a religion is born. I guess I've seen too many born again preachers and politicians caught in motels with young boys and young girls who were not related to them or each other, to swallow the whole woo-woo pill in one sitting.

I feel now that I am a Certified Yoga Teacher I will have to re-classify myself nearer to the top of the woo-woo food chain and star using the word Guru in front of my name as I experienced in Hawaii. A young women who called herself Guru Diana, charged twenty bucks for Yoga at our timeshare, brought her jewelry and tapes, and flyers for her upcoming retreats and took us through all of four poses, all sitting postures, and all nearly worthless. I guess in every trade there are charlatans, I just don't want to be one. I am now going to start believing that I am a Guru. After all if Trump can suggest something as stupid as arming teachers, I may as well be confident in my divinity. Arming teachers will only result in more shootings of Principals. ,There is my first premonition. Revelations 1. On a serious note these rituals and ceremonies honor the best in us and the hard work that has gone into achieving something of meaning. It is time I took these things seriously and not matter of factly. The things I am blessed to do and achieve are only dreams for some and I had better begin to understand that.

When I started drum circles at my church an older man, 84 years, named Don who was a retired businessman, and who held a top spot with Westinghouse, came up to me after drumming one day. He said to me, "I want to thank you for starting this drumming, this is the first time in my life I have touched an instrument." I was shocked and didn't know what to say. I hugged him said thank you, and could feel tears running down my cheek. For me being a long time professional drummer, drum circles were no big deal, and I dismissively organized them. But what was not that important to me was greatly important to someone else and I try to always remember that. The things I have been blessed to be able to do, I no longer take lightly, but give thanks and have gratitude, because that could change in a second.

--If we have one hand in yesterday, and one in tomorrow, we have no hands to hold on to today-----

The shuttle we had hired to take us away from Uvita, since some of us had planes to catch that day, Friday, left at 2:30 heading for Jaco where I would be dropped off. My flight was not until Monday morning the 26th, since to leave Saturday or Sunday would have cost 200$ more. I decided to spend the night again in the same hotel. Hotel Cadillac Rock, with the life size cutout of the Beatles on the porch roof. The hotel was next to the Beatle Bar, which was, I found out that evening, the local pick-up bar for White Western men to meet and leave with the local tradeswomen of the night. Since prostitution was not a crime in this country, business was good. After working on this book for nearly three hours straight I decided to get dressed and go next door for a soda. When I walked in the Beatle Bar, I thought there was a wedding going on, all the women in black gowns, but in short order found out what the real party was about. I was approached right away by a couple of Ticos (natives) and asked if I would like a massage. Of course I would always like a massage but I knew what they were thinking. This was not my first rodeo, but I acted flattered and surprised. I was surprised at how chubby most of them were for girls relying on body image to sell their wares. This however didn't keep the swinging doors shut as cab after cab dropped off and picked up. I got tired of the show and was exhausted since I was up at 5 to prepare for my class and bid my new friends a good night. I never had ill feeling toward ladies or men of the night since it takes a fairly strong ego to stay in the ring after many rejections, and still put on a happy face. I guess we all do things for money that we would rather not, like work, and this is just another avenue, connecting to the same street. The beeping cab horns all night were the biggest irritant.

I had to make my way to San Jose today on my next stop homeward. I asked the lady at the hotel where the bus terminal to san Jose was here in Jaco. She pointed up the street and said "Three meters" I thought she must have said three miles or three minutes so I had them call me a cab since I had a huge suitcase packed for three weeks of living and another bag and a knapsack. I lugged my stuff downstairs and the cab came, he loaded my stuff, went to the end of the block and stopped to let me off and unload! I astonishingly hollered "No this can't be the place!" He literally drove me 100 ft. and charged me three colonies, about 5 USD. WTF, was my first thought but he did what I asked. I was the stupid one for not figuring out how far it really was. Actually I couldn't have rolled my stuff that far in any event, so I quit bitching. I was trying to stay in my "accept everything as it is "stage. The bus ticket window didn't open till noon and the bus didn't leave until 1 pm. So I waited a half hour to buy the ticket and sat on a high curb with all the other mostly Ticos, in the shade, thankfully, but in the heat and humidity none the less. We all sat there, fifty of us waiting for the bus. Although there is plenty of mass transit in Costa Rica there is not much money spent on Bus terminals or waiting areas for passengers, except for the terminal in Uvita and San Jose. The rest of them look like something out of "Grapes of Wrath" or simply roadside stands. I expected to see Clint Eastwood with a large piece of grass sticking out his mouth walk by and say "Hey Mister why ya' sittin' in the heat, where do you think you are Costa Rica?"

The two hour ride dragged as they all do in a bus, but I was out of the bus and in my new motel in less than three hours since I left Jaco, that was not bad.

The place I chose to spend Saturday night is a cute little boutique hotel one block from the first hotel, Casa Roland, Where I stayed the first night I arrived. At that time while I was walking around I noticed another hotel named Colours Oasis. It flew the rainbow flag so I walked in and got a tour around. This is a gorgeous and artfully planned hotel with a roof top sundeck an inground , indoor sort of, pool, and plenty of places to sit and chat or chill. I paid 60$ for a night and couldn't have been happier. I went this morning to say goodbye to Ana the cook at the Roland whom I met when I stayed there. I gave her a hug, showed her my Yoga certificate, and bid her farewell, since she was in the middle of cooking breakfast for their guests, and had no time to chat. My next, and final stop was a "Yoga Nature Preserve" hotel close to the airport which was my goal since I have to be at the airport tomorrow at 5:30. The exact name is Flor de Mayo Airport Nature preserve. I will leave here at noon and arrive there in twenty minutes or so. This too was a fairly inexpensive stay coming in at 79$ including tax. They display a line of yoga mats along the pool in their online website so I'll be curious to know what that is about. I felt fortunate to have found so many cool places to stay so far from home but the places I chose certainly were a feast for the eyes, so small and so cute.

-------Not all is what it appears----

My Yoga hotel near the airport turns out to be the home of Carol the daughter of the folks who came here many years ago to save the macaws. That giant parrot like creature you see sitting on a pirates shoulder. Apparently they were endangered and in many cases wounded, and her parents bought this lovely spacious property somewhat close to the airport, but far from anything else, like dinner. Luckily, since it is pouring outside now, I earlier bought two pastries that will now be my sustenance until morning. This place looks a little creepy, kind of a cross between the Adams Family house and the Ponderosa. Carol appears to be one of those hold-over Hippies who probably grows bean sprouts in jars, is gluten free, eats organics and cage free eggs, washes with Castile soap, rolls her own joints and refuses to shave her arm pits. But I could be guessing. I have been here almost three hours and haven't gone out of my room. Her boyfriend looks astonishingly like the guitar player in my band forty years ago, who, when I told him he was tuning up too much between songs, ripped the entire bridge holding the strings, right off the guitar.

Of course this was not him, but I was freaked. I'm pretty much out of travel money now and I did pay her for the room. I feel a poor review coming on but things may change once I leave my room and actually talk to them. This may turn out to be a pleasant experience? She booked this as a

Nature Preserve, but I can see that it is closer to something out of The Hobbits. The pool shown in the online booking is unusable, and THAT is more of a nature preserve, harboring numerous species of toads, frogs and other things with tails. To see the rest of the property one has to meander down a road on the side of the property and go down a hill etc. but having given away my snake boots to Julio, I'm probably going to stay in my bedroom and listen to it rain.

Being from Phoenix hearing rain is like seeing Big Foot, it happens a few times every decade, so listening to the warm rain is very soothing as I sit here and write this. But before I continue I'm going to go out and meet them and see if I can go a little way out into the yard and report back honestly.

"Offering a pool, spa, and wellness center." Their ad reads. I just returned from walking the grounds here and while it is close to the airport, the host tried to talk me into having them drive me for twenty bucks when it is normally a five dollar trip by taxi. "But taxi's won't come here." She commented. I can see why. Native people here are still very superstitious and are probably frightened to enter the grounds. There is no pool I could find, no deck with lovely people doing yoga, as in their ad, and no wellness center. However I am not going to let this ruin an otherwise good vacation. In twelve hours I will be at the airport, and on my way home. In the end I will be asked to give a review for Booking .com and payback, as they say, is a bitch .This trip was an amazing adventure, one I'll never forget with people I'll never forget doing the best they can to find spiritual identity and advance personal growth by voluntarily giving up creature comforts to reach beyond and into something deeper inside themselves. I had a whole new outlook at least toward my wife. We had never been apart this long nor have I ever taken a vacation this long in all my working life. When I got home I looked at my wife and after a little smooching, noticed how much of her beauty I had been either ignoring or overlooking. She is very attractive and sexy and we made love like never before the night I returned. I guess mindfulness works! One of the teachers told me that of twenty people she interviewed, only two told her they were actually going to teach yoga, and that they had embarked on this journey for personal growth. I get that. I am more stoked now about teaching yoga than I was before, since my knowledge of yoga overall has been vastly expanded. For eight years all I knew was the same 26 postures that Bikram Yoga does over and over and over. That practice kept me in shape logging 1600 classes in 8 yrs, but left me out of the wider loop that is Yoga. It is like being given a Japanese ham sandwich for 8 years and then finding out there are Chinese buffets!

I have an urge now to try my teaching skills on the yoga public and see how long it takes me to feel comfortable doing this. I like yoga and they say find what you like and find a way to make money at it and you will be happy. I believe that is true.

I'm not sure how long it will take me to stop throwing toilet paper in the trash can, as they do all over Costa Rica, but I'll probably enjoy flushing it away the first couple of times. This country has a magical flare to it, even the air is full of aromatic smells, brought about by the multitude of flowering plants everywhere you look. I have never seen more gorgeous beaches in my life, even Hawaii can't compare, in my opinion. I will miss this place, no doubt, but something keeps telling me that I'll be back. Not sure when or what for, but I will be back. I will return.

I went over my trip with my spiritual advisor for many hours on the phone this afternoon and I asked her, if after all she had heard from me, "Do you think I'm enlightened?"

"My dear boy", I could see her smile even over the phone. " You've been enlightened since the day you were born and then you were covered by the trappings of this world, so that the enlightenment was covered and afraid to shine through. Find that happy little boy that used to smile with eager anticipation at everything new, and be excited at the promise of each new day. Be grateful for a beautiful body and good health. Treat your body like the temple it is and it will treat you like the heavenly body you are. You don't need to add things like knowledge, money, and things of this world to feel your worth. You need to peel away the onion and divest yourself of those things that no longer serve you, things that keep you hidden from the desires of your heart. Your heart knows what you want, your brain tries to make you fit in. Happiness lies only in your self-acceptance. Your enlightenment is a fact, with which I will not quarrel."

I was so happy to hear that, and there was a long pause on the phone.

"So what do you think I should do now?" I asked her.

" My dear boy, keep doing what you've always done."

"Chop wood, and carry water."

Namaste

NOTES